Lean Cuisine: A Comprehensive Guide to Sustainable Weight Loss and Delicious Recipes:

Achieve Your Ideal Weight with Proven Strategies and Mouthwatering Meals

Doris J Adam's

Copyright © 2024 by Doris J. Adam's

Table of Contents:

1. Introduction

Sarah had struggled with her weight for years. Despite trying various diets and exercise plans, she found herself stuck in a cycle of losing weight only to gain it back again. Frustrated and disheartened, she was about to give up hope of ever achieving her weight loss goals.

One day, Sarah stumbled upon a book titled "Lean Cuisine: A Comprehensive Guide to Sustainable Weight Loss and Delicious Recipes." Intrigued by the promise of sustainable weight loss and mouthwatering meals, she decided to give it a chance.

As Sarah delved into the book, she was pleasantly surprised by the wealth of information it contained. From understanding the science of weight loss to practical tips for meal planning and preparation, the book provided her with the knowledge she needed to make lasting changes to her lifestyle.

Armed with the guidance from the book, Sarah began to implement small changes in her diet and exercise routine. She started incorporating more fruits and vegetables into her meals, practicing portion control, and engaging in regular physical activity that she enjoyed.

What truly made a difference for Sarah was the delicious recipes included in the book. She discovered new and exciting ways to prepare healthy meals that were both satisfying and nutritious. From hearty breakfasts to flavorful dinners and guilt-free snacks, the recipes kept her motivated and excited about her weight loss journey.

Over time, Sarah began to see significant progress. Not only was she losing weight, but she also felt more energetic, confident, and empowered. With each passing week, she celebrated new milestones and accomplishments, knowing that she was finally on the right path to achieving her goals.

Months later, Sarah had transformed both physically and mentally. Thanks to the guidance and support of "Lean Cuisine," she had not only lost weight but had also adopted a healthier and more balanced lifestyle that she could maintain for the long term. As she closed the book one final time, she felt grateful for the positive impact it had made on her life.

2. Understanding Weight Loss:

Losing weight is often perceived as a simple equation of consuming fewer calories than you expend. However, the process of weight loss is far more complex and multifaceted. It involves a combination of factors including diet, exercise, metabolism, genetics, and even psychological aspects.

At its core, weight loss occurs when the body burns more calories than it takes in, leading to a calorie deficit. This deficit can be achieved through reducing calorie intake, increasing physical activity, or ideally, a combination of both. However, the quality of the calories consumed and the type of physical activity performed also play crucial roles in determining the effectiveness and sustainability of weight loss efforts.

Moreover, understanding the science behind weight loss is essential for making informed decisions about diet and exercise. For example, certain foods may have different effects on hunger, metabolism, and energy levels, making it important to choose nutrient-dense options that support satiety and overall health.

Additionally, factors such as hormone levels, sleep quality, stress levels, and even gut health can influence weight loss outcomes. Addressing these factors and adopting a holistic approach to health and wellness can significantly enhance the success of weight loss efforts and contribute to long-term success.

Ultimately, understanding weight loss goes beyond simply counting calories or following a strict diet plan. It involves gaining insight into how the body responds to various foods and activities, identifying personal barriers and triggers, and developing sustainable habits that promote overall well-being. By taking a comprehensive and informed approach to weight loss, individuals can achieve their goals and maintain a healthy lifestyle for the long term.

The Science of Weight Loss:

Weight loss is a complex physiological process governed by the principles of energy balance and metabolism. At its core, weight loss occurs when the body expends more energy (calories) than it consumes, resulting in a calorie deficit. This deficit triggers the body to utilize stored fat as a source of fuel, leading to a reduction in body weight over time.

Several key factors influence the body's ability to lose weight effectively:

Caloric Intake and Expenditure: The fundamental principle of weight loss revolves around creating a calorie deficit. This can be achieved by consuming fewer calories through diet or increasing energy expenditure through physical activity.

Metabolism: Metabolism refers to the complex biochemical processes that occur within the body to maintain life. Basal metabolic rate (BMR) accounts for the majority of energy expenditure and is influenced by factors such as age, gender, body composition, and genetics. Understanding one's metabolic rate is crucial for optimizing weight loss efforts.

Macronutrient Balance: The composition of one's diet, including the balance of carbohydrates, proteins, and fats, can impact weight loss outcomes. For example, protein-rich foods can promote feelings of fullness and preserve lean muscle mass during calorie restriction, while carbohydrates provide energy for physical activity.

Hormonal Regulation: Hormones play a significant role in regulating appetite, metabolism, and fat storage. Hormones such as insulin, leptin, ghrelin, and cortisol influence hunger levels, energy expenditure, and the body's response to food intake. Imbalances in hormone levels can impede weight loss progress and may need to be addressed through dietary and lifestyle modifications.

Nutrient Density: Choosing nutrient-dense foods that are rich in vitamins, minerals, and antioxidants can support overall health and facilitate weight loss. These foods provide essential nutrients while minimizing empty calories, leading to greater satiety and improved metabolic function.

Behavioral and Psychological Factors: Psychological factors such as stress, emotional eating, and food cravings can impact dietary choices and adherence to weight loss plans. Addressing these behaviors through strategies such as mindfulness, stress management, and behavior modification techniques is essential for long-term success.

By understanding the underlying science of weight loss, individuals can make informed decisions about diet, exercise, and lifestyle habits that support their goals.

Adopting a holistic approach that takes into account the interplay of various physiological and psychological factors can lead to sustainable weight loss and improved overall health and well-being.

Setting Realistic Goals:

Setting realistic goals is a crucial first step on the journey to successful weight loss. While it's natural to feel motivated and eager to achieve dramatic results quickly, setting overly ambitious or unrealistic goals can lead to frustration, disappointment, and ultimately, derailment of your efforts. Instead, focusing on setting achievable and sustainable goals is key to long-term success.

Here are some key principles to keep in mind when setting realistic weight loss goals:

Be Specific: Define your goals with clarity and precision. Rather than simply aiming to "lose weight," specify how much weight you want to lose and by when. For example, setting a goal to lose 1-2 pounds per week is more specific and achievable than aiming to lose 20 pounds in a month.

Be Realistic: Consider your starting point, lifestyle, and personal circumstances when setting goals. While it's tempting to aspire to rapid weight loss, aim for a rate of weight loss that is realistic and sustainable over the long term. Rapid weight loss can often be unsustainable and may lead to health complications or rebound weight gain.

Break it Down: Break your overarching weight loss goal into smaller, more manageable milestones. Celebrating incremental progress along the way can help maintain motivation and momentum. For example, if your ultimate goal is to lose 50 pounds, set smaller milestones of 5 or 10 pounds at a time.

Consider Non-Scale Victories: Remember that weight loss is not the only measure of success. Consider setting goals related to other aspects of health and well-being, such as improved energy levels, increased physical fitness, or better sleep quality. Non-scale victories can provide additional motivation and reinforce positive lifestyle changes.

Focus on Behavior Changes: Instead of solely focusing on outcomes, such as the number on the scale, concentrate on the behaviors and habits that will support your weight loss goals. For example, setting goals related to increasing physical activity, reducing portion sizes, or cooking more meals at home can contribute to long-term success.

Adjust as Needed: Be flexible and willing to adjust your goals as you progress. Life circumstances, plateaus, and unexpected challenges may require reassessment and modification of your goals. Remember that setbacks are a natural part of the journey, and it's important to stay adaptable and resilient.

By setting realistic and achievable goals, you set yourself up for success on your weight loss journey. Embrace the process, celebrate your progress, and focus on making sustainable lifestyle changes that support your long-term health and well-being.

Overcoming Common Challenges in Weight Loss:

Embarking on a weight loss journey can be both rewarding and challenging. Along the way, many individuals encounter common obstacles that can hinder progress and test their resolve. However, with the right mindset and strategies, these challenges can be overcome, paving the way for success. Here are some common challenges in weight loss and how to overcome them:

Plateaus: It's not uncommon to reach a point where weight loss stalls, despite continued efforts. Plateaus can be frustrating, but they are a normal part of the process. To overcome plateaus, consider adjusting your calorie intake, increasing physical activity, varying your exercise routine, or incorporating more nutrient-dense foods into your diet. Remember to stay patient and trust the process – persistence pays off.

Cravings and Temptations: Cravings for unhealthy foods and temptations to indulge in high-calorie treats can derail even the most well-intentioned weight loss efforts. To overcome cravings, try practicing mindfulness techniques, such as deep breathing or distraction strategies. Additionally, keep tempting foods out of sight and stock your kitchen with nutritious alternatives. Planning ahead and having healthy snacks on hand can help you resist the urge to give in to temptation.

Emotional Eating: Many people turn to food for comfort or as a coping mechanism during times of stress, boredom, or emotional distress. Recognizing triggers for emotional eating and finding alternative ways to manage emotions can help break this cycle. Engage in stress-relieving activities such as exercise, meditation, or spending time with loved ones. Seek support from friends, family, or a therapist if emotional eating becomes a significant challenge.

Social Pressures and Peer Influence: Social situations, such as gatherings, parties, and dining out, can present challenges for sticking to a healthy eating plan. Communicate your goals to friends and family members and enlist their support in making healthier choices. When dining out, scan the menu beforehand, choose options that align with your goals, and practice portion control. Remember that it's okay to indulge occasionally, but aim to make balanced choices overall.

Time Constraints and Busy Schedules: Busy lifestyles can make it difficult to prioritize healthy eating and exercise. However, with careful planning and time management, it's possible to incorporate healthy habits into even the busiest of schedules. Schedule workouts into your calendar, prepare meals and snacks ahead of time, and prioritize self-care activities. Remember that consistency is key, even if it means squeezing in shorter workouts or opting for quick and nutritious meal options.

Lack of Motivation or Accountability: Maintaining motivation and accountability can be challenging, especially when progress is slow or setbacks occur. Find sources of inspiration, whether it's setting rewards for reaching milestones, joining a support group or online community, or working with a coach or accountability partner. Keep track of your progress, celebrate achievements, and remind yourself of the reasons why you embarked on your weight loss journey in the first place.

By acknowledging and proactively addressing common challenges, you can navigate obstacles more effectively and stay on track towards your weight loss goals. Remember to be patient and kind to yourself, and celebrate each small victory along the way. With perseverance and determination, you can overcome challenges and achieve lasting success in your weight loss journey.

3. Creating a Balanced Diet Plan:

A balanced diet plan is essential for supporting weight loss goals while ensuring that your body receives the nutrients it needs for optimal health and well-being. A well-rounded diet provides a variety of nutrients, including carbohydrates, proteins, fats, vitamins, and minerals, in appropriate proportions. Here are some key principles for creating a balanced diet plan:

Include a Variety of Foods: Aim to include a wide variety of foods from all food groups in your diet. This includes fruits, vegetables, whole grains, lean proteins, and healthy fats. Each food group provides essential nutrients that contribute to overall health and can help satisfy hunger and prevent feelings of deprivation.

Focus on Whole, Unprocessed Foods: Choose whole, minimally processed foods whenever possible. Whole foods are typically rich in nutrients, fiber, and antioxidants, and they tend to be more filling and satisfying than highly processed alternatives. Incorporate plenty of fruits, vegetables, whole grains, lean meats, fish, nuts, seeds, and legumes into your meals and snacks.

Watch Portion Sizes: Pay attention to portion sizes to avoid overeating and to ensure that you're consuming an appropriate number of calories for your goals. Use tools such as measuring cups, food scales, or visual cues to help gauge appropriate portion sizes. Focus on eating until you feel satisfied, rather than overly full.

Balance Macronutrients: Each meal should contain a balance of carbohydrates, proteins, and fats to provide sustained energy and promote feelings of fullness. Aim to include sources of lean protein (such as chicken, turkey, fish, tofu, or legumes), complex carbohydrates (such as whole grains, fruits, and vegetables), and healthy fats (such as avocados, nuts, seeds, and olive oil) in each meal.

Moderate Sugar and Processed Foods: Limit the intake of added sugars, refined grains, and processed foods, as these can contribute excess calories and offer little nutritional value. Choose whole, natural sources of sweetness, such as fruit, and opt for whole grains over refined grains whenever possible.

Stay Hydrated: Hydration is essential for overall health and can support weight loss by promoting satiety and preventing dehydration-related hunger cues. Aim to drink plenty of water throughout the day and limit sugary beverages and alcohol.

Plan Ahead and Be Flexible: Take time to plan your meals and snacks in advance to ensure that you have nutritious options available when hunger strikes. However, be flexible and willing to adapt your plan as needed based on changing circumstances or preferences. Listen to your body's hunger and fullness cues and adjust your intake accordingly.

By following these principles and creating a balanced diet plan that incorporates a variety of nutrient-dense foods, you can support your weight loss goals while nourishing your body and promoting overall health and well-being. Remember that consistency and moderation are key, and aim for progress, not perfection, on your journey towards a healthier lifestyle.

Building a Nutrient-Rich Plate:

Creating a nutrient-rich plate is an essential component of a balanced diet plan and can support your weight loss goals by providing the body with the vital nutrients it needs for optimal health and energy. A nutrient-rich plate incorporates a variety of foods from different food groups to ensure a diverse array of vitamins, minerals, antioxidants, and macronutrients. Here's how to build a nutrient-rich plate:

Fill Half Your Plate with Fruits and Vegetables: Fruits and vegetables are rich in vitamins, minerals, fiber, and antioxidants, making them essential components of a nutrient-rich plate. Aim to fill half of your plate with colorful, non-starchy vegetables such as leafy greens, broccoli, bell peppers, carrots, and tomatoes. Incorporate a variety of fruits into your meals and snacks for added flavor and nutrition.

Add Lean Protein: Protein is important for supporting muscle growth, repair, and satiety. Choose lean sources of protein such as chicken, turkey, fish, tofu, tempeh, legumes, or low-fat dairy products. Aim to include a palm-sized portion of protein on your plate to help balance blood sugar levels and promote feelings of fullness.

Incorporate Whole Grains: Whole grains provide complex carbohydrates, fiber, and essential nutrients such as B vitamins and minerals. Choose whole grains such as brown rice, quinoa, barley, oats, whole wheat pasta, or whole grain bread to add texture and satiety to your meals. Aim to fill about a quarter of your plate with whole grains.

Include Healthy Fats: Healthy fats are essential for supporting brain health, hormone production, and nutrient absorption. Incorporate sources of healthy fats such as avocados, nuts, seeds, olive oil, and fatty fish like salmon or trout into your meals. Use these fats in moderation to add flavor and richness to your plate.

Be Mindful of Portions: Pay attention to portion sizes to avoid overeating and to ensure that you're consuming an appropriate balance of nutrients. Use visual cues such as your hand or a measuring tool to gauge portion sizes for different food groups. Remember that it's okay to enjoy a variety of foods in moderation, but aim for balance and variety overall.

Hydrate with Water: Water is essential for overall health and can support weight loss by promoting hydration and satiety. Drink water throughout the day and with meals to stay hydrated and to help control hunger cues. Limit sugary beverages and alcohol, which can contribute excess calories and offer little nutritional value.

By building a nutrient-rich plate that incorporates a variety of colorful fruits and vegetables, lean proteins, whole grains, and healthy fats, you can support your weight loss goals while nourishing your body with the essential nutrients it needs for optimal health and well-being. Aim for balance, variety, and moderation in your dietary choices, and enjoy the benefits of a nutrient-rich diet.

Portion Control Techniques:

Portion control is a key component of weight loss and maintaining a healthy diet. By managing portion sizes, you can enjoy a wide variety of foods while still controlling calorie intake and promoting weight loss. Here are some effective portion control techniques to help you manage your portions and support your weight loss goals:

Use Smaller Plates and Bowls: Opt for smaller plates and bowls to help control portion sizes visually. Research has shown that people tend to eat larger portions when served on larger plates, so downsizing your dinnerware can help you eat less without feeling deprived.

Measure Portions: Use measuring cups, spoons, or a food scale to accurately measure portions of foods, especially when cooking or serving yourself. This can help you become more aware of appropriate portion sizes and prevent overeating. Pay attention to recommended serving sizes on food labels to guide your portion control efforts.

Divide Your Plate: Use the "plate method" to divide your plate into sections for different food groups. Fill half of your plate with non-starchy vegetables, one-quarter with lean protein, and one-quarter with whole grains or starchy vegetables. This balanced approach ensures that you're getting a variety of nutrients while controlling portion sizes.

Practice Mindful Eating: Pay attention to hunger and fullness cues and eat slowly to give your body time to register satisfaction. Put down your fork between bites, chew food thoroughly, and savor the flavors and textures of each bite. Avoid distractions such as television or smartphones while eating, as this can lead to mindless overeating.

Pre-Portion Snacks: Instead of eating directly from the package, portion out snacks into individual servings to prevent mindless munching. Divide larger packages of snacks into smaller, single-serving containers or bags to make it easier to grab a controlled portion when hunger strikes.

Be Strategic with Treats: Enjoying treats and indulgences in moderation is an important part of a balanced diet. Instead of eliminating your favorite foods entirely, practice portion control by enjoying smaller servings of treats occasionally. Use smaller dessert plates or bowls to serve yourself, and savor each bite slowly to fully enjoy the experience.

Listen to Your Body: Pay attention to hunger and fullness signals and stop eating when you feel satisfied, rather than overly full. Tune in to how your body feels before, during, and after meals, and adjust portion sizes accordingly. Remember that it's okay to leave food on your plate if you're no longer hungry, even if there are leftovers.

By incorporating these portion control techniques into your daily routine, you can manage your portions effectively, support your weight loss goals, and develop healthier eating habits for the long term. Experiment with different strategies to find what works best for you, and remember that small changes can add up to significant results over time.

Building Smart Snacking Strategies:

Snacking can be an important part of a healthy diet, providing energy between meals and preventing overeating at mealtimes. However, it's essential to choose nutrient-rich snacks that support your weight loss goals and promote overall health. Here are some smart snacking strategies to help you make healthier choices and avoid mindless munching:

Plan Ahead: Take time to plan your snacks in advance, just like you would with meals. Keep a variety of healthy snacks on hand at home, at work, or on the go, so you're less likely to reach for unhealthy options when hunger strikes. Pre-portion snacks into individual servings to prevent overeating.

Choose Nutrient-Dense Options: Opt for snacks that are rich in nutrients, such as fruits, vegetables, whole grains, lean proteins, and healthy fats. These foods provide essential vitamins, minerals, fiber, and protein, while keeping calories in check. Examples of nutrient-dense snacks include apple slices with nut butter, Greek yogurt with berries, raw vegetables with hummus, or a small handful of nuts and seeds.

Mind Your Portions: Be mindful of portion sizes when snacking to avoid consuming excess calories. Use small bowls or containers to serve yourself snacks, rather than eating directly from the package. Stick to single-serving portions to prevent mindless munching and overeating.

Pair Protein with Fiber: Combining protein and fiber in your snacks can help keep you feeling full and satisfied between meals. Protein-rich snacks such as Greek yogurt, cottage cheese, hard-boiled eggs, or edamame paired with high-fiber foods like fruits, vegetables, or whole grains make for a filling and nutritious snack option.

Snack with Purpose: Instead of snacking out of boredom, stress, or habit, tune in to your hunger cues and snack with purpose. Ask yourself if you're truly hungry or if you're eating out of other reasons. Choose snacks that satisfy hunger and provide sustained energy, rather than empty calories or sugary treats.

Hydrate: Sometimes, feelings of hunger can be mistaken for thirst. Stay hydrated throughout the day by drinking plenty of water, herbal tea, or infused water. Before reaching for a snack, try drinking a glass of water first to see if your hunger subsides.

Practice Portion Control: If you're craving a less nutritious snack, such as chips, cookies, or chocolate, practice portion control by enjoying a small serving rather than indulging in the entire package. Put a handful of chips or a few cookies on a plate and savor each bite slowly, rather than mindlessly snacking straight from the bag.

Listen to Your Body: Pay attention to how your body responds to different snacks and adjust your choices accordingly. Choose snacks that make you feel energized, satisfied, and nourished, rather than sluggish or guilty. Honor your hunger and fullness cues and stop eating when you feel satisfied.

By incorporating these smart snacking strategies into your daily routine, you can make healthier choices, support your weight loss goals, and maintain energy levels throughout the day. Experiment with different snack options and find what works best for you, and remember that snacking can be an enjoyable and satisfying part of a balanced diet.

4. Exercise and Fitness:

Exercise is a crucial component of a healthy lifestyle and plays a significant role in supporting weight loss, improving physical fitness, and enhancing overall well-being. Whether you're aiming to shed pounds, build muscle, or simply boost your mood, incorporating regular physical activity into your routine offers numerous benefits. Here's how exercise and fitness can contribute to your health and weight loss goals:

Calorie Burn and Weight Loss: One of the primary benefits of exercise for weight loss is its ability to increase calorie expenditure. Engaging in physical activity helps burn calories, creating a calorie deficit when combined with a balanced diet. Both aerobic exercise (such as walking, running, cycling, or swimming) and strength training (such as weightlifting or bodyweight exercises) can contribute to weight loss by burning calories and building lean muscle mass.

Improves Metabolic Health: Regular exercise can improve metabolic health by increasing insulin sensitivity, reducing blood sugar levels, and lowering risk factors for chronic diseases such as type 2 diabetes and cardiovascular disease. Exercise also helps regulate hormones involved in appetite control, leading to better weight management and reduced risk of obesity-related conditions.

Increases Muscle Strength and Endurance: Strength training exercises help build and maintain muscle mass, which is essential for increasing metabolism, supporting joint health, and enhancing functional strength and mobility. Incorporating resistance training into your workout routine can help improve muscle tone, increase bone density, and reduce the risk of age-related muscle loss (sarcopenia).

Boosts Mood and Mental Health: Exercise has powerful mood-boosting effects and can help alleviate symptoms of stress, anxiety, and depression. Physical activity stimulates the release of endorphins, neurotransmitters that promote feelings of happiness and well-being. Regular exercise also improves sleep quality, reduces feelings of fatigue, and enhances cognitive function, leading to better overall mental health and resilience.

Enhances Cardiovascular Health: Aerobic exercise strengthens the heart and lungs, improves circulation, and enhances cardiovascular endurance. Regular cardiovascular exercise helps lower blood pressure, reduce LDL (bad) cholesterol levels, and increase HDL (good) cholesterol levels, lowering the risk of heart disease and stroke.

Supports Long-Term Weight Maintenance: Beyond weight loss, exercise plays a critical role in maintaining weight loss and preventing weight regain over time. Incorporating regular physical activity into your lifestyle helps sustain metabolic rate, preserve lean muscle mass, and promote healthier eating habits, making it easier to maintain a lower weight in the long term.

Promotes Overall Well-Being: Exercise offers numerous benefits beyond physical health, including improved mood, increased energy levels, better sleep, and enhanced quality of life. Regular physical activity provides a sense of accomplishment, boosts self-confidence, and fosters social connections when done in group settings or with workout buddies.

Incorporating a combination of aerobic exercise, strength training, flexibility, and balance exercises into your weekly routine can help you reap the full range of benefits that exercise and fitness have to offer. Aim for at least 150 minutes of moderate-intensity aerobic activity or 75 minutes of vigorous-intensity aerobic activity per week, along with two or more days of strength training exercises targeting all major muscle groups. Remember to start gradually, listen to your body, and choose activities that you enjoy to make exercise a sustainable and enjoyable part of your lifestyle.

Incorporating Physical Activity into Your Routine:

Regular physical activity is essential for maintaining overall health, supporting weight loss efforts, and improving quality of life. However, finding the time and motivation to exercise can be challenging amidst busy schedules and competing priorities. Fortunately, there are many strategies you can use to incorporate physical activity into your daily routine, making it easier to stay active and reap the benefits of exercise. Here are some tips for incorporating physical activity into your routine:

Set Realistic Goals: Start by setting realistic and achievable goals for physical activity. Whether it's aiming to exercise for a certain number of minutes per day or completing a specific workout routine, having clear goals can help keep you focused and motivated.

Find Activities You Enjoy: Choose activities that you enjoy and look forward to doing. Whether it's walking, jogging, cycling, dancing, swimming, or playing sports, finding activities that you find enjoyable makes it easier to stay committed and motivated over the long term.

Schedule Exercise Time: Treat exercise like any other important appointment or commitment by scheduling it into your daily calendar. Choose a time of day that works best for you, whether it's first thing in the morning, during your lunch break, or in the evening after work. Consistency is key, so aim to stick to your scheduled exercise times as much as possible.

Break it Up: If finding time for a long workout seems daunting, break it up into shorter bouts of activity throughout the day. Aim for at least 10 minutes of moderate-intensity activity at a time, such as taking a brisk walk during your coffee break or doing a quick workout during commercial breaks while watching TV.

Incorporate Activity into Daily Tasks: Look for opportunities to sneak in extra physical activity throughout your day. Take the stairs instead of the elevator, park farther away from your destination, or walk or bike to run errands whenever possible. Incorporating activity into your daily tasks can add up to significant calorie expenditure over time.

Make it Social: Exercise with friends, family members, or coworkers to make it more enjoyable and social. Join a fitness class, sports team, or walking group, or simply invite a friend to join you for a workout. Exercising with others can provide accountability, motivation, and social support, making it more likely that you'll stick to your routine.

Use Technology: Take advantage of technology to track your activity levels, set goals, and stay motivated. Use fitness apps, activity trackers, or wearable devices to monitor your progress, set reminders, and track your workouts. Many apps and devices offer features such as guided workouts, social challenges, and rewards for meeting activity goals.

Be Flexible: Be willing to adapt your exercise routine based on changing circumstances or priorities. If you're short on time or unable to do your usual workout, find alternative ways to stay active, such as doing a quick bodyweight workout at home or taking a walk during your lunch break.

Incorporating physical activity into your routine doesn't have to be overwhelming or time-consuming. By setting realistic goals, choosing activities you enjoy, scheduling exercise time, breaking it up into shorter bouts, incorporating activity into daily tasks, making it social, using technology, and staying flexible, you can make exercise a regular and enjoyable part of your lifestyle. Remember that every little bit of activity adds up, so find ways to move your body in ways that feel good and work for you.

Effective Workouts for Weight Loss:

When it comes to weight loss, incorporating regular exercise into your routine is crucial for burning calories, building muscle, and boosting metabolism. While any form of physical activity can contribute to weight loss, certain types of workouts are particularly effective at torching calories and promoting fat loss. Here are some effective workouts for weight loss:

Cardiovascular Exercise: Cardiovascular or aerobic exercise is one of the most effective forms of exercise for burning calories and promoting weight loss. Activities such as walking, running, cycling, swimming, dancing, and jumping rope elevate your heart rate and increase calorie expenditure. Aim for at least 150 minutes of moderate-intensity aerobic exercise or 75 minutes of vigorous-intensity aerobic exercise per week to support weight loss goals.

High-Intensity Interval Training (HIIT): HIIT involves alternating between short bursts of intense exercise and periods of rest or lower-intensity activity. This form of exercise has been shown to be highly effective for burning calories, boosting metabolism, and promoting fat loss in a shorter amount of time compared to steady-state cardio. HIIT workouts can include exercises such as sprints, burpees, jumping jacks, and mountain climbers performed at maximum effort for 20-30 seconds followed by short rest periods.

Strength Training: Strength training or resistance training is essential for building and maintaining lean muscle mass, which is important for increasing metabolism and promoting fat loss. Incorporating strength training exercises such as weightlifting, bodyweight exercises, resistance band exercises, or using weight machines helps to sculpt and tone your muscles while burning calories. Aim to include strength training exercises targeting all major muscle groups at least two days per week.

Circuit Training: Circuit training combines cardiovascular exercise with strength training in a high-intensity, interval-based format. It involves moving quickly between different exercises with minimal rest between sets, effectively challenging both the cardiovascular and muscular systems. Circuit training workouts can include a combination of bodyweight exercises, resistance exercises, and cardio intervals, making it a time-efficient and effective way to burn calories and promote weight loss.

Group Fitness Classes: Group fitness classes offer a motivating and social environment for getting active and burning calories. Classes such as indoor cycling, kickboxing, boot camp, Zumba, or circuit training provide structured workouts led by certified instructors, helping to keep you accountable and motivated. Group classes also offer variety and can challenge your body in new ways, preventing workout plateaus and boredom.

Outdoor Activities: Take advantage of outdoor activities such as hiking, trail running, biking, or swimming for a fun and effective way to burn calories and enjoy the great outdoors. Outdoor activities provide opportunities for varying terrain and intensity levels, making them ideal for challenging your body and promoting weight loss.

Flexibility and Mobility Work: Don't overlook the importance of flexibility and mobility work in your workout routine. Incorporating activities such as yoga, Pilates, or stretching helps improve flexibility, range of motion, and joint health, reducing the risk of injury and enhancing overall physical performance. These activities also promote relaxation, stress reduction, and mindfulness, which are important for overall well-being.

When designing a workout routine for weight loss, aim for a combination of cardiovascular exercise, strength training, and flexibility work to achieve balanced results. Remember to gradually increase intensity and duration as your fitness level improves, and always listen to your body and prioritize safety. With consistency, determination, and the right mix of workouts, you can achieve your weight loss goals and enjoy the many benefits of regular exercise.

Staying Motivated and Consistent:

Maintaining motivation and consistency is key to achieving your weight loss and fitness goals. While getting started may feel exciting and energizing, staying committed to your routine over the long term can be challenging. However, with the right strategies and mindset, you can overcome obstacles and stay on track towards success. Here are some tips for staying motivated and consistent on your journey:

Set Clear, Achievable Goals: Define specific, measurable, and achievable goals that provide direction and purpose for your efforts. Whether it's losing a certain amount of weight, improving fitness levels, or fitting into a certain clothing size, having clear goals gives you something to work towards and helps keep you focused.

Find Your Why: Identify your reasons for wanting to lose weight or get fit, and connect with your deeper motivations. Whether it's improving your health, boosting confidence, setting a positive example for your loved ones, or simply feeling better in your own skin, having a strong "why" can help fuel your determination and keep you committed when the going gets tough.

Celebrate Progress: Celebrate your achievements and milestones along the way, no matter how small they may seem. Recognize and acknowledge your progress, whether it's reaching a new fitness milestone, sticking to your workout routine for a certain number of days, or making healthier food choices. Celebrating progress helps reinforce positive behaviors and boosts confidence and motivation.

Find What You Enjoy: Choose activities and exercises that you genuinely enjoy and look forward to doing. Whether it's dancing, hiking, swimming, yoga, or playing sports, finding activities that bring you joy makes it easier to stay motivated and consistent. Experiment with different types of workouts until you find what resonates with you, and don't be afraid to try new things.

Mix It Up: Keep your workouts fresh and exciting by varying your routine and trying different activities and exercises. Incorporate a mix of cardiovascular exercise, strength training, flexibility work, and recreational activities to prevent boredom and challenge your body in new ways. Mixing up your routine also prevents plateaus and keeps you engaged and motivated.

Create a Support System: Surround yourself with a supportive network of friends, family members, or workout buddies who encourage and motivate you along the way. Share your goals with others, join fitness communities or social media groups, or enlist the help of a workout partner or accountability buddy to keep you motivated and accountable.

Track Your Progress: Keep track of your workouts, nutrition, and progress over time to monitor your success and stay accountable. Use a workout journal, fitness app, or wearable device to track metrics such as workouts completed, calories burned, steps taken, or inches lost. Seeing tangible evidence of your progress can provide motivation and reinforce your commitment to your goals.

Practice Self-Compassion: Be kind to yourself and practice self-compassion, especially during challenging times or setbacks. Understand that progress is not always linear, and there will be ups and downs along the way. Instead of beating yourself up over missed workouts or slip-ups in your nutrition, focus on what you can control in the present moment and keep moving forward with renewed determination.

Visualize Success: Visualize yourself achieving your goals and imagine how it will feel to accomplish what you've set out to do. Create a mental image of your future self and focus on the positive emotions associated with reaching your goals. Visualization techniques can help reinforce your motivation and keep you focused on your desired outcome.

Practice Consistency: Consistency is key to long-term success, so prioritize making small, sustainable changes to your habits and routines. Focus on building healthy habits one step at a time and commit to showing up for yourself consistently, even on days when you don't feel like it. Remember that every positive choice you make brings you one step closer to your goals.

By incorporating these strategies into your daily life, you can stay motivated and consistent on your weight loss and fitness journey. Remember that progress takes time and patience, so be kind to yourself and stay focused on the bigger picture. With dedication, perseverance, and a positive mindset, you can achieve your goals and create lasting changes for a healthier, happier life.

5. Practicing Mindful Eating Habits:

Mindful eating is a practice that involves paying attention to the sensory experience of eating and being fully present in the moment. By cultivating awareness around your eating habits, thoughts, and sensations, you can develop a healthier relationship with food, improve digestion, and make more conscious choices about what and how much you eat. Here are some tips for incorporating mindful eating habits into your daily life:

Eat Without Distractions: Minimize distractions during meals by turning off the TV, putting away electronic devices, and focusing solely on the act of eating. Avoid eating while working, scrolling through social media, or multitasking, as this can lead to mindless eating and overconsumption.

Savor Each Bite: Take the time to truly savor and enjoy each bite of food, paying attention to the taste, texture, and aroma. Chew your food slowly and mindfully, allowing yourself to fully experience the flavors and sensations. Eating slowly gives your body time to register feelings of fullness, reducing the likelihood of overeating.

Listen to Your Body: Tune in to your body's hunger and fullness cues and eat in response to physical hunger rather than emotional or external triggers. Before eating, ask yourself if you're truly hungry or if you're eating out of boredom, stress, or habit. Stop eating when you feel satisfied, even if there is food left on your plate.

Practice Gratitude: Cultivate gratitude for the food you're eating by taking a moment to acknowledge where it came from, how it was prepared, and the nourishment it provides for your body. Express gratitude for the abundance of food available to you and the effort that went into bringing it to your table.

Engage Your Senses: Engage all of your senses while eating, not just taste. Notice the colors, shapes, and textures of your food, as well as the sounds it makes as you chew. Pay attention to the temperature and how the food feels in your mouth. Engaging your senses can enhance your enjoyment of food and help you feel more satisfied.

Be Mindful of Portion Sizes: Be mindful of portion sizes and serve yourself appropriate amounts of food based on your hunger and satiety cues. Use smaller plates and bowls to help control portion sizes visually, and avoid eating directly from large containers or packages, as this can lead to mindless overeating.

Practice Non-Judgment: Approach eating with a non-judgmental attitude and without guilt or shame. Recognize that all foods can fit into a balanced diet, and there are no "good" or "bad" foods. Instead of labeling foods as off-limits, focus on making balanced choices and enjoying everything in moderation.

Stay Present: Bring your attention back to the present moment whenever your mind starts to wander or you find yourself eating on autopilot. Practice mindfulness techniques such as deep breathing, body scans, or gentle stretching before meals to center yourself and cultivate awareness.

Reflect on Your Choices: After eating, take a moment to reflect on how you feel physically and emotionally. Notice any patterns or triggers that may influence your eating habits and consider how you can make more conscious choices in the future. Reflecting on your eating experiences can help you learn more about yourself and your relationship with food.

By incorporating mindful eating habits into your daily routine, you can develop a healthier relationship with food, improve digestion, and make more conscious choices about what and how much you eat. Remember that mindful eating is a practice that takes time and patience to cultivate, so be gentle with yourself and approach it with curiosity and openness. As you become more attuned to your body's cues and sensations, you'll discover a greater sense of satisfaction and enjoyment in your eating experiences.

Managing Emotional Eating:

Emotional eating is a common behavior characterized by consuming food in response to emotional cues rather than physical hunger. Many people turn to food for comfort, stress relief, boredom, or to cope with difficult emotions such as sadness, anxiety, loneliness, or frustration. While occasional emotional eating is normal and can provide temporary relief, relying on food as a primary coping mechanism can lead to unhealthy eating habits, weight gain, and negative emotions surrounding food and body image.

There are several factors that contribute to emotional eating, including:

Stress: Stress is one of the most common triggers for emotional eating. During times of stress, the body releases cortisol, a hormone that can increase appetite and cravings for high-calorie, comfort foods. Many people turn to food as a way to cope with stress and soothe their emotions.

Boredom: Feelings of boredom or monotony can lead to mindless eating as a way to pass the time or add excitement to dull moments. Without other stimulating activities to engage in, food may become a default source of entertainment or distraction.

Loneliness and Isolation: Feelings of loneliness or social isolation can trigger emotional eating as a way to fill an emotional void or seek comfort. Sharing a meal with others is often associated with feelings of connection and belonging, and eating alone may exacerbate feelings of loneliness.

Negative Emotions: Unpleasant emotions such as sadness, anxiety, anger, or frustration can lead to emotional eating as a way to numb or suppress uncomfortable feelings. Food may provide a temporary distraction or sense of relief from emotional pain.

Habitual Patterns: Over time, certain behaviors and routines become ingrained as habits, including the habit of turning to food in response to emotions. These automatic eating patterns can be difficult to break, even when they no longer serve a helpful purpose.

While emotional eating can provide temporary comfort or relief, it often leads to feelings of guilt, shame, and regret afterward. Additionally, relying on food as a coping mechanism can contribute to weight gain, poor nutrition, and negative emotions surrounding body image and self-esteem.

Managing emotional eating involves developing healthier coping strategies and learning to respond to emotions in ways that don't involve food. Some strategies for managing emotional eating include:

Identifying Triggers: Pay attention to the situations, emotions, and thoughts that trigger your urge to eat emotionally. Keeping a food diary or journal can help you identify patterns and recognize your triggers more easily.

Finding Alternative Coping Strategies: Instead of turning to food for comfort, explore alternative coping strategies such as deep breathing, meditation, journaling, or engaging in hobbies or activities you enjoy.

Practicing Mindful Eating: Cultivate mindfulness and awareness around your eating habits by paying attention to your thoughts, feelings, and sensations before, during, and after eating. Practice mindful eating techniques such as eating slowly, chewing your food thoroughly, and savoring each bite.

Seeking Support: Reach out to friends, family members, or professionals who can offer support, encouragement, and guidance as you work to overcome emotional eating patterns. Talking to others about your struggles can provide validation and perspective.

Addressing Underlying Emotions: Instead of suppressing or avoiding difficult emotions, practice acknowledging and processing them in healthy ways. Seek support from a therapist or counselor if needed to work through underlying emotional issues.

By developing awareness around emotional eating patterns, finding alternative coping strategies, practicing mindfulness, seeking support, and addressing underlying emotions, you can learn to manage emotional eating more effectively and develop a healthier relationship with food and your emotions. Remember that progress takes time and patience, so be gentle with yourself as you navigate this journey toward greater emotional well-being.

Developing a Healthy Relationship with Food:

A healthy relationship with food is characterized by balanced eating habits, positive attitudes towards food and body image, and a mindful approach to nourishing both the body and mind. Cultivating a healthy relationship with food involves fostering self-awareness, practicing self-compassion, and adopting behaviors that promote physical and emotional well-being. Here are some key principles for developing a healthy relationship with food:

Listen to Your Body: Tune in to your body's hunger and fullness cues and eat in response to physical hunger rather than external or emotional triggers. Pay attention to how different foods make you feel and honor your cravings while also recognizing when you're satisfied.

Eat Mindfully: Practice mindful eating by savoring each bite, chewing slowly, and paying attention to the sensory experience of eating. Be present in the moment and avoid distractions such as TV, phones, or computers while eating. By being mindful, you can better enjoy your meals and develop a deeper appreciation for food.

Ditch the Diet Mentality: Let go of restrictive dieting behaviors and adopt a more flexible and intuitive approach to eating. Focus on nourishing your body with a variety of whole, nutrient-dense foods rather than labeling foods as "good" or "bad." Allow yourself to enjoy treats in moderation without guilt or shame.

Cultivate Self-Compassion: Practice self-compassion and kindness towards yourself, especially when it comes to food and body image. Treat yourself with the same empathy and understanding that you would offer to a friend facing similar challenges. Be gentle with yourself during times of struggle and remember that nobody is perfect.

Challenge Negative Thoughts: Challenge negative thoughts and beliefs about food, body image, and weight. Recognize that your worth is not determined by your appearance or what you eat. Focus on positive affirmations and self-talk that promote self-acceptance and body positivity.

Find Joy in Cooking and Eating: Rediscover the joy of cooking and eating by exploring new recipes, flavors, and cuisines. Experiment with fresh, whole ingredients and involve friends or family members in meal preparation and sharing. Embrace food as a source of pleasure and nourishment rather than a source of stress or anxiety.

Practice Moderation: Embrace a balanced approach to eating that includes a wide variety of foods in moderation. Allow yourself to enjoy all foods in moderation, including indulgent treats, while also prioritizing nutrient-rich whole foods that nourish your body. Strive for balance, not perfection, in your eating habits.

Stay Active and Engaged: Stay physically active and engaged in activities that bring you joy and fulfillment beyond eating. Find hobbies, interests, and social connections that provide meaning and fulfillment in your life, reducing the reliance on food for emotional fulfillment.

Seek Support if Needed: If you struggle with disordered eating patterns or negative body image, seek support from a therapist, counselor, or registered dietitian who specializes in eating disorders or intuitive eating. Professional guidance can provide personalized strategies and resources to help you heal your relationship with food and your body.

Be Patient and Persistent: Developing a healthy relationship with food is a journey that takes time and patience. Be patient with yourself as you navigate this process and celebrate the progress you make along the way. Remember that small, consistent changes can lead to significant improvements in your relationship with food and your overall well-being.

By practicing self-awareness, mindfulness, self-compassion, and moderation, you can develop a healthier relationship with food that nourishes both your body and soul. Remember that food is not just fuel; it's also a source of pleasure, connection, and cultural heritage. Embrace a balanced approach to eating that honors your body's needs while also allowing for enjoyment and flexibility. With time, patience, and self-compassion, you can cultivate a positive and empowering relationship with food that supports your health and happiness for years to come.

6. Meal Planning and Preparation:

Meal planning and preparation are essential components of a healthy and balanced lifestyle. By taking the time to plan and prepare nutritious meals ahead of time, you can save time, money, and energy while also making it easier to stick to your health and wellness goals. Whether you're looking to lose weight, improve your eating habits, or simply eat more mindfully, meal planning and preparation can help you achieve success. Here's how to get started:

Set Aside Time for Planning: Dedicate a specific day each week to plan your meals for the upcoming week. Set aside some time to review your schedule, consider your dietary preferences and nutritional goals, and create a meal plan that works for you. Having a plan in place can help reduce stress and decision-making throughout the week.

Create a Weekly Menu: Use your meal plan to create a weekly menu that includes breakfasts, lunches, dinners, and snacks for each day. Consider factors such as convenience, variety, and balance when selecting recipes and meals. Aim for a mix of protein, healthy fats, complex carbohydrates, and fiber-rich fruits and vegetables in each meal.

Make a Shopping List: Once you have your menu planned out, create a shopping list of all the ingredients you'll need for the week. Check your pantry, refrigerator, and freezer to see what ingredients you already have on hand, and make note of what you need to buy. Stick to your list while grocery shopping to avoid impulse purchases and ensure you have everything you need for your meals.

Prep Ingredients in Advance: Take some time to prep ingredients in advance to streamline meal preparation during the week. Wash and chop fruits and vegetables, cook grains and proteins, and portion out snacks and ingredients for recipes ahead of time. Storing prepped ingredients in airtight containers or resealable bags makes it easy to assemble meals quickly and efficiently.

Batch Cook: Consider batch cooking large quantities of staple ingredients such as grains, beans, proteins, and sauces to use in multiple meals throughout the week. Cook once and enjoy the benefits of having ready-made components that can be mixed and matched to create a variety of meals.

Use Time-Saving Kitchen Tools: Invest in time-saving kitchen tools and appliances that can help simplify meal preparation. Tools such as a slow cooker, Instant Pot, food processor, or spiralizer can save you time and effort in the kitchen while allowing you to create delicious and nutritious meals with ease.

Store Meals Properly: Store prepared meals and ingredients properly to maintain freshness and quality throughout the week. Use airtight containers, reusable storage bags, or meal prep containers to store individual portions of meals in the refrigerator or freezer. Label containers with the date and contents for easy identification.

Stay Flexible: Be flexible and adaptable with your meal plan and preparation routine. Life can be unpredictable, and you may need to adjust your plans based on changes in schedule, unexpected events, or ingredient availability. Embrace flexibility and make modifications as needed to accommodate shifting priorities and preferences.

Enjoy the Process: Approach meal planning and preparation as an opportunity to nourish yourself and your loved ones with delicious and nutritious food. Enjoy the process of cooking and experimenting with new recipes, flavors, and ingredients. Get creative in the kitchen and have fun exploring different cuisines and cooking techniques.

Evaluate and Adjust: Take time at the end of each week to evaluate how your meal plan and preparation routine worked for you. Reflect on what went well, what could be improved, and any adjustments you'd like to make for the following week. Use feedback from your experience to refine your approach and create a meal plan that better meets your needs and preferences.

By incorporating meal planning and preparation into your routine, you can streamline your eating habits, save time and money, and make healthier choices more accessible and convenient. With a little bit of planning and preparation, you can set yourself up for success and enjoy the benefits of nourishing meals that support your health and well-being.

Tips for Successful Meal Planning:

Meal planning is a valuable tool for saving time, money, and stress while also promoting healthier eating habits. By taking the time to plan your meals ahead of time, you can streamline your grocery shopping, reduce food waste, and ensure that you have nutritious and delicious meals ready to go throughout the week. Here are some tips for successful meal planning:

Set Realistic Goals: Start by setting realistic and achievable goals for your meal planning efforts. Consider factors such as your schedule, dietary preferences, budget, and cooking skills when setting goals. Start small and gradually build upon your successes as you become more comfortable with meal planning.

Know Your Schedule: Take inventory of your weekly schedule, including work commitments, appointments, and social activities, to determine how much time you'll have for meal preparation and cooking. Adjust your meal plan accordingly, opting for quick and easy meals on busy days and more elaborate recipes when you have more time available.

Create a Master List of Recipes: Compile a list of your favorite recipes, including breakfasts, lunches, dinners, and snacks, to serve as inspiration for your meal plan. Organize your recipes by category (e.g., chicken, vegetarian, pasta) to make it easier to choose meals that fit your preferences and dietary needs.

Plan Your Meals Weekly or Biweekly: Choose a specific day each week or every other week to sit down and plan your meals for the upcoming period. Use a meal planning template or calendar to map out your meals for each day, including breakfasts, lunches, dinners, and snacks. Be sure to account for leftovers and any meals eaten outside of the home.

Consider Balance and Variety: Aim for balance and variety in your meal plan by including a mix of protein, healthy fats, complex carbohydrates, and fiber-rich fruits and vegetables in each meal. Rotate through different protein sources (e.g., chicken, fish, beans, tofu) and experiment with new ingredients and flavors to keep meals interesting.

Use Theme Nights or Rotations: Simplify meal planning by assigning theme nights or rotations to different days of the week. For example, you could have "Meatless Monday," "Taco Tuesday," "Soup and Salad Wednesday," and so on. Having a framework in place can make it easier to choose meals and ensure variety throughout the week.

Shop with a Plan: Use your meal plan to create a shopping list of all the ingredients you'll need for the week. Check your pantry, refrigerator, and freezer to see what ingredients you already have on hand, and make note of what you need to buy. Stick to your list while grocery shopping to avoid impulse purchases and ensure you have everything you need for your meals.

Prep Ingredients in Advance: Take some time to prep ingredients in advance to streamline meal preparation during the week. Wash and chop fruits and vegetables, cook grains and proteins, and portion out snacks and ingredients for recipes ahead of time. Storing prepped ingredients in airtight containers or resealable bags makes it easy to assemble meals quickly and efficiently.

Be Flexible and Adaptive: Be flexible and adaptive with your meal plan, recognizing that life can be unpredictable. Embrace flexibility and make adjustments to your meal plan as needed based on changes in schedule, unexpected events, or ingredient availability. Having a plan in place provides structure, but it's important to be willing to adapt as circumstances change.

Batch Cook and Freeze Meals: Take advantage of batch cooking to prepare larger quantities of meals or components that can be frozen and enjoyed later. Cook soups, stews, casseroles, and other freezer-friendly meals in bulk and portion them out into individual servings for quick and convenient meals on busy days.

Plan for Leftovers: Embrace leftovers as a time-saving strategy by intentionally cooking extra portions to enjoy as leftovers for future meals. Plan for leftovers by incorporating them into your meal plan or repurposing them into new dishes to prevent food waste and save time and effort in the kitchen.

Review and Reflect: Take time at the end of each week to review how your meal plan worked for you. Reflect on what went well, what could be improved, and any adjustments you'd like to make for the following week. Use feedback from your experience to refine your approach and create a meal plan that better meets your needs and preferences.

By incorporating these tips into your meal planning routine, you can save time, money, and stress while also enjoying delicious and nutritious meals that support your health and well-being. With a little bit of planning and preparation, you can set yourself up for success and make mealtime a more enjoyable and satisfying experience.

Time-Saving Meal Prep Techniques:

Meal prep is a valuable strategy for saving time, reducing stress, and ensuring that you have healthy and delicious meals ready to enjoy throughout the week. By dedicating a few hours to meal prep each week, you can streamline your cooking process, minimize last-minute meal decisions, and make it easier to stick to your health and nutrition goals. Here are some time-saving meal prep techniques to help you get started:

Plan Your Menu in Advance: Before you begin meal prepping, take some time to plan your menu for the week ahead. Choose recipes that are simple, easy to prepare in bulk, and can be easily reheated or assembled during the week. Consider factors such as variety, balance, and nutritional content when selecting recipes.

Batch Cook Staple Ingredients: Streamline your meal prep process by batch cooking staple ingredients that can be used in multiple meals throughout the week. Cook large quantities of grains (such as rice, quinoa, or pasta), proteins (such as chicken, tofu, or beans), and roasted vegetables to use as the building blocks for various meals.

Prep Ingredients in Bulk: Wash, chop, and prepare fruits, vegetables, and other ingredients in bulk to save time during meal prep. Use a food processor or mandoline slicer to quickly chop vegetables, and portion out ingredients into resealable containers or bags for easy access throughout the week.

Utilize Slow Cooker or Instant Pot: Take advantage of slow cookers or Instant Pots to prepare hands-off meals that require minimal effort. Simply add ingredients to the pot in the morning, set the timer, and let the appliance do the work while you go about your day. Slow-cooked meals such as soups, stews, and chili are perfect for batch cooking and can be portioned out for multiple meals.

Make One-Pot or Sheet Pan Meals: Simplify meal prep by opting for one-pot or sheet pan meals that require minimal cleanup. Choose recipes that allow you to cook everything in a single pot or on a sheet pan, reducing the number of dishes and pans you need to wash afterward. These meals are also great for batch cooking and can be easily reheated throughout the week.

Portion Out Meals in Advance: Once your meals are cooked and prepared, portion them out into individual containers or meal prep containers for easy storage and grab-and-go convenience. Label containers with the name of the dish and the date it was prepared to keep track of freshness and ensure food safety.

Freeze Meals for Later Use: Take advantage of your freezer to store prepped meals for later use. Portion out meals into freezer-safe containers or resealable bags and label them with the name of the dish and the date it was prepared. Frozen meals can be reheated quickly in the microwave or oven for a convenient meal option when you're short on time.

Prep Breakfast and Snacks: Don't forget to prep breakfast and snacks as part of your meal prep routine. Prepare grab-and-go options such as overnight oats, yogurt parfaits, energy balls, or pre-portioned snacks like nuts, fruits, and vegetables to have on hand throughout the week.

Clean as You Go: To minimize cleanup time after meal prep, clean as you go by washing dishes, wiping down countertops, and putting away ingredients as you finish using them. This will help keep your kitchen organized and tidy throughout the meal prep process.

Stay Organized: Keep your meal prep session organized by setting up a designated workspace with all the necessary tools, utensils, and ingredients within reach. Use clear containers or labels to identify prepped ingredients and meals, making it easy to find what you need during the week.

By incorporating these time-saving meal prep techniques into your routine, you can simplify your cooking process, save time and energy, and enjoy delicious and nutritious meals throughout the week. With a little bit of planning and preparation, you can set yourself up for success and make mealtime a more enjoyable and stress-free experience.

Budget-Friendly Shopping Strategies:

Managing your grocery budget effectively is key to maintaining a healthy and balanced diet without overspending. With the right strategies in place, you can stretch your food dollars further while still enjoying nutritious and delicious meals. Here are some budget-friendly shopping strategies to help you make the most of your grocery budget:

Create a Meal Plan: Start by creating a weekly or biweekly meal plan that outlines the meals you'll be cooking and eating throughout the week. Plan your meals around ingredients you already have on hand and incorporate affordable staples such as grains, beans, and seasonal produce.

Shop with a List: Before heading to the grocery store, make a list of all the items you need for your planned meals as well as any household essentials. Stick to your list while shopping to avoid impulse purchases and ensure you only buy what you need.

Set a Budget: Establish a weekly or monthly grocery budget based on your household income and expenses. Divide your budget into categories such as groceries, household items, and non-food essentials, and track your spending to stay within your budgetary limits.

Compare Prices and Shop Sales: Take advantage of sales, discounts, and promotions to save money on your grocery purchases. Compare prices between different brands and store options to find the best deals on the items you need. Look for sales flyers, digital coupons, and loyalty programs to maximize your savings.

Buy in Bulk: Purchase pantry staples such as grains, beans, rice, pasta, and canned goods in bulk to save money over time. Buying in bulk often offers a lower cost per unit and reduces packaging waste. Consider investing in a membership to a warehouse club or shopping at bulk food stores for additional savings.

Choose Generic or Store Brands: Opt for generic or store brands over name-brand products to save money without sacrificing quality. Many generic products are comparable in taste and quality to their name-brand counterparts but come at a lower price point. Compare labels and ingredients to ensure you're getting the best value for your money.

Shop Seasonally and Locally: Purchase fruits and vegetables that are in season to take advantage of lower prices and better quality. Visit local farmers' markets or participate in community-supported agriculture (CSA) programs to access fresh, locally grown produce at affordable prices. Buying seasonal and local produce also supports local farmers and reduces environmental impact.

Minimize Food Waste: Reduce food waste by planning meals that use up ingredients you already have on hand and incorporating leftovers into future meals. Store perishable items properly to extend their shelf life, and use up ingredients before they spoil. Get creative with leftovers by repurposing them into new dishes or incorporating them into soups, salads, or stir-fries.

Consider Frozen and Canned Options: Explore frozen and canned options for fruits, vegetables, and proteins, which often offer similar nutritional value to fresh counterparts at a lower cost. Stock up on frozen vegetables, berries, and seafood when they're on sale, and choose canned beans, tomatoes, and other pantry staples for convenience and affordability.

Plan for Meatless Meals: Incorporate meatless meals into your meal plan to save money on groceries and promote plant-based eating. Choose budget-friendly protein sources such as beans, lentils, tofu, eggs, and dairy products to replace or supplement meat in recipes. Experiment with vegetarian and vegan recipes to discover new flavors and culinary traditions.

Avoid Shopping When Hungry: To prevent impulse purchases and overspending, avoid shopping on an empty stomach. Eat a snack or meal before heading to the grocery store to curb cravings and stick to your shopping list.

Pack Your Own Snacks and Beverages: Save money on snacks and beverages by packing your own instead of purchasing them on the go. Prepare homemade snacks such as trail mix, granola bars, fruit, and vegetable sticks to take with you when you're out and about. Bring a reusable water bottle to stay hydrated without relying on expensive bottled beverages.

By implementing these budget-friendly shopping strategies, you can stretch your grocery budget further, reduce food waste, and enjoy nutritious and satisfying meals without breaking the bank. With careful planning and mindful spending, you can make the most of your food dollars and achieve your health and wellness goals within your budgetary constraints.

7. Delicious and Nutritious Recipes:

Eating healthy doesn't mean sacrificing flavor or satisfaction. With the right ingredients and cooking techniques, you can create delicious and nutritious meals that nourish your body and delight your taste buds. Whether you're cooking for yourself, your family, or entertaining guests, these recipes are sure to please even the most discerning palates:

Quinoa and Black Bean Stuffed Bell Peppers:

Ingredients:
4 bell peppers, any color
1 cup quinoa, rinsed
1 can black beans, drained and rinsed
1 cup corn kernels (fresh or frozen)
1 cup diced tomatoes
1 teaspoon cumin
1 teaspoon chili powder
Salt and pepper to taste
Instructions:
Preheat the oven to 375°F (190°C). Cut the tops off the bell peppers and remove the seeds and membranes.
In a medium saucepan, bring 2 cups of water to a boil. Add the quinoa, reduce heat to low, cover, and simmer for 15-20 minutes, or until the quinoa is cooked and water is absorbed.

In a large mixing bowl, combine the cooked quinoa, black beans, corn, diced tomatoes, cumin, chili powder, salt, and pepper. Mix well.
Stuff each bell pepper with the quinoa mixture, pressing down gently to pack it in.
Place the stuffed peppers in a baking dish and cover with foil. Bake in the preheated oven for 25-30 minutes, or until the peppers are tender.
Serve hot, garnished with chopped cilantro or avocado slices if desired.
Mediterranean Chickpea Salad:

Ingredients:
2 cans chickpeas, drained and rinsed
1 cucumber, diced
1 cup cherry tomatoes, halved
1/2 red onion, thinly sliced
1/4 cup Kalamata olives, pitted and halved
1/4 cup crumbled feta cheese (optional)
2 tablespoons fresh lemon juice
2 tablespoons extra virgin olive oil
1 teaspoon dried oregano
Salt and pepper to taste
Instructions:
In a large mixing bowl, combine the chickpeas, cucumber, cherry tomatoes, red onion, and Kalamata olives.
In a small bowl, whisk together the lemon juice, olive oil, dried oregano, salt, and pepper to make the dressing.
Pour the dressing over the chickpea mixture and toss to coat evenly.

Sprinkle the crumbled feta cheese on top, if using, and toss gently to combine.

Serve immediately or refrigerate for at least 30 minutes to allow the flavors to meld before serving.

Sheet Pan Lemon Herb Salmon and Vegetables:

Ingredients:
4 salmon fillets
1 pound baby potatoes, halved
2 cups broccoli florets
1 cup cherry tomatoes
2 tablespoons olive oil
2 tablespoons fresh lemon juice
2 cloves garlic, minced
1 teaspoon dried thyme
1 teaspoon dried rosemary
Salt and pepper to taste
Instructions:
Preheat the oven to 400°F (200°C). Line a large baking sheet with parchment paper or aluminum foil.

Place the salmon fillets in the center of the baking sheet and arrange the baby potatoes, broccoli, and cherry tomatoes around them.

In a small bowl, whisk together the olive oil, lemon juice, minced garlic, dried thyme, dried rosemary, salt, and pepper to make the marinade.

Pour the marinade over the salmon and vegetables, tossing gently to coat everything evenly.

Arrange the ingredients in a single layer on the baking sheet, making sure the salmon fillets are skin-side down.

Bake in the preheated oven for 15-20 minutes, or until the salmon is cooked through and the vegetables are tender.

Serve hot, garnished with fresh herbs or lemon slices if desired.

These recipes are just a starting point for creating delicious and nutritious meals that you and your family will love. Feel free to customize them with your favorite ingredients and flavors to suit your tastes and dietary preferences. With a little creativity and experimentation, you can enjoy healthy and satisfying meals every day of the week.

Breakfasts to Start Your Day Right:

Breakfast is often hailed as the most important meal of the day, and for good reason. A nutritious breakfast provides the fuel and nutrients your body needs to kickstart your metabolism, boost your energy levels, and set a positive tone for the day ahead. From quick and easy options for busy mornings to leisurely weekend brunch ideas, here are some breakfasts to start your day right:

Overnight Oats:

Overnight oats are a convenient and customizable breakfast option that can be prepared the night before and enjoyed cold or heated up in the morning. Simply combine rolled oats with your choice of milk (such as almond milk, coconut milk, or dairy milk), Greek yogurt, and toppings such as fresh fruit, nuts, seeds, and sweeteners like honey or maple syrup. Let the mixture soak in the refrigerator overnight, and wake up to a delicious and nutritious breakfast ready to enjoy.
Avocado Toast:

Avocado toast is a simple yet satisfying breakfast option that can be customized with a variety of toppings to suit your tastes. Start with a slice of whole-grain bread or toast and spread mashed avocado on top. Add toppings

such as sliced tomatoes, poached eggs, smoked salmon, crumbled feta cheese, arugula, or a sprinkle of Everything Bagel seasoning for extra flavor and nutrition.
Greek Yogurt Parfait:

Greek yogurt parfaits are a delicious and protein-rich breakfast option that can be assembled in minutes. Layer Greek yogurt with granola, fresh berries, sliced bananas, and a drizzle of honey or maple syrup in a glass or bowl for a nutritious and satisfying morning meal. Customize your parfait with additional toppings such as nuts, seeds, dried fruit, or coconut flakes for added texture and flavor.
Vegetable Omelette:

Start your day with a hearty and satisfying vegetable omelette packed with protein and fiber. Whisk together eggs with a splash of milk or water and season with salt and pepper. Pour the egg mixture into a heated non-stick skillet and cook until set, then add your favorite vegetables such as spinach, bell peppers, onions, mushrooms, and tomatoes. Fold the omelette in half and serve with a side of whole-grain toast or a mixed greens salad for a complete breakfast.
Smoothie Bowl:

Smoothie bowls are a refreshing and nutritious breakfast option that can be customized with your favorite fruits, vegetables, and toppings. Blend together frozen fruit such as bananas, berries, mango, or pineapple with

Greek yogurt, spinach or kale, and a splash of milk or juice until smooth and creamy. Pour the smoothie into a bowl and top with granola, sliced fruit, shredded coconut, chia seeds, and a drizzle of nut butter or honey for added texture and flavor.

Whole-Grain Pancakes or Waffles:

Treat yourself to a stack of whole-grain pancakes or waffles topped with fresh fruit, Greek yogurt, and a drizzle of pure maple syrup for a wholesome and satisfying breakfast. Make a batch of pancakes or waffles ahead of time and freeze them for quick and easy breakfasts during the week. Experiment with different flavors and add-ins such as cinnamon, vanilla extract, mashed banana, or chocolate chips for variety.

Egg and Veggie Breakfast Burritos:

Prepare a batch of hearty breakfast burritos filled with scrambled eggs, sautéed vegetables, black beans, and shredded cheese wrapped in whole-grain tortillas. Make a large batch ahead of time and freeze them individually for a convenient grab-and-go breakfast option. Serve with salsa, avocado slices, and Greek yogurt or sour cream for dipping.

Chia Seed Pudding:

Chia seed pudding is a nutritious and satisfying breakfast option that can be prepared in advance and enjoyed cold or heated up in the morning. Mix together chia seeds with your choice of milk (such as almond milk, coconut milk, or dairy milk) and sweetener (such as honey, maple syrup, or agave nectar) in a jar or bowl. Let the mixture sit in the refrigerator overnight to thicken, then top with fresh fruit, nuts, seeds, or granola before serving.

These breakfast ideas are not only delicious and satisfying but also provide a good balance of macronutrients to fuel your body and brain for the day ahead. Whether you prefer sweet or savory, quick and easy or leisurely and indulgent, there's a breakfast option to suit every taste and lifestyle. By starting your day with a nutritious and satisfying meal, you'll set yourself up for success and feel energized and focused throughout the day.

Energizing Lunch Ideas:

A nutritious and energizing lunch is essential for powering through the rest of your day with focus and vitality. Whether you're working, studying, or running errands, a well-balanced lunch can provide the fuel your body needs to sustain energy levels and stay productive. Here are some energizing lunch ideas to keep you fueled and satisfied:

Grilled Chicken and Quinoa Salad:

Toss together grilled chicken breast slices, cooked quinoa, mixed greens, cherry tomatoes, cucumber slices, avocado chunks, and crumbled feta cheese in a large bowl. Drizzle with a homemade vinaigrette made with olive oil, lemon juice, Dijon mustard, and honey for added flavor. This protein-packed salad is both satisfying and energizing, providing a balance of lean protein, whole grains, and fresh vegetables to keep you feeling full and focused throughout the afternoon.
Salmon and Avocado Sushi Bowls:

Whip up a batch of sushi rice and divide it among bowls. Top each bowl with cooked salmon fillet chunks, sliced avocado, cucumber strips, shredded carrots, and edamame beans. Drizzle with soy sauce, sesame oil, and sriracha for a burst of flavor. These sushi bowls are rich in omega-3 fatty acids, healthy fats, and fiber, providing long-lasting energy and supporting brain health.

Mediterranean Chickpea Wrap:

Spread hummus on a whole-grain tortilla and layer with cooked chickpeas, sliced cucumber, cherry tomatoes, red onion, Kalamata olives, crumbled feta cheese, and fresh parsley. Roll up the tortilla and slice it in half for a portable and satisfying lunch option. This Mediterranean-inspired wrap is packed with fiber, protein, and vitamins, making it a nutritious and energizing choice for busy days.

Quinoa and Black Bean Stuffed Sweet Potatoes:

Bake sweet potatoes until tender, then slice them open and fluff the flesh with a fork. Fill each sweet potato with a mixture of cooked quinoa, black beans, diced bell peppers, corn kernels, chopped cilantro, and a squeeze of lime juice. Top with a dollop of Greek yogurt or avocado slices for added creaminess. These stuffed sweet potatoes are a hearty and satisfying lunch option that provides a good balance of complex carbohydrates, plant-based protein, and fiber to keep you feeling full and energized.

Asian-Inspired Noodle Salad:

Cook soba noodles according to package instructions and rinse under cold water. Toss the noodles with thinly sliced red cabbage, shredded carrots, snap peas, bell peppers, green onions, and chopped cilantro in a large

bowl. Drizzle with a homemade dressing made with soy sauce, sesame oil, rice vinegar, ginger, and garlic for a burst of flavor. This refreshing noodle salad is packed with vegetables and whole grains, providing a boost of energy without weighing you down.
Chickpea and Vegetable Stir-Fry:

Sauté diced onion, garlic, ginger, bell peppers, broccoli florets, and snap peas in a wok or skillet until tender-crisp. Add cooked chickpeas and stir-fry sauce (made with soy sauce, hoisin sauce, sesame oil, and rice vinegar) to the pan and toss to coat. Serve the stir-fry over cooked brown rice or quinoa for a filling and nutritious lunch option that's packed with protein, fiber, and vitamins.
Turkey and Hummus Wrap:

Spread hummus on a whole-grain wrap and layer with sliced turkey breast, spinach leaves, shredded carrots, cucumber strips, and roasted red peppers. Roll up the wrap tightly and slice it in half for a satisfying and protein-rich lunch option. Pair it with a side of fresh fruit or vegetable sticks and hummus for added nutrients and energy.
Vegetable and Lentil Soup:

Make a batch of hearty vegetable and lentil soup using a variety of vegetables such as carrots, celery, onions, tomatoes, and spinach, along with cooked lentils and vegetable broth. Season with herbs and spices such as thyme, oregano, cumin, and paprika for extra flavor.

Enjoy a bowl of soup with a slice of whole-grain bread or a side salad for a nourishing and comforting lunch that will keep you warm and satisfied.

These energizing lunch ideas are not only delicious and satisfying but also provide the nutrients and energy your body needs to stay focused and productive throughout the day. With a little bit of planning and preparation, you can enjoy nutritious and flavorful lunches that power you through even the busiest of days.

Satisfying Dinners for Weight Loss:

Dinner is an important meal of the day, especially when you're trying to lose weight. It's essential to choose satisfying meals that keep you full and satisfied while also supporting your weight loss goals. Here are some delicious and nutritious dinner ideas that are perfect for helping you shed pounds without sacrificing flavor or satisfaction:

Grilled Lemon Herb Chicken with Roasted Vegetables:

Marinate chicken breasts in a mixture of fresh lemon juice, minced garlic, olive oil, and herbs such as thyme, rosemary, and oregano. Grill the chicken until cooked through and juicy. Serve with a side of roasted vegetables such as carrots, broccoli, and Brussels sprouts tossed with olive oil, salt, and pepper. This protein-packed dinner is low in calories and high in fiber, vitamins, and minerals, making it a satisfying and nutritious option for weight loss.
Baked Salmon with Asparagus and Quinoa:

Season salmon fillets with salt, pepper, and a squeeze of lemon juice. Bake in the oven until flaky and tender. Meanwhile, steam or roast asparagus spears until crisp-tender. Serve the baked salmon with a side of cooked quinoa and steamed asparagus for a balanced and satisfying dinner. Salmon is rich in omega-3 fatty acids, which support heart health and promote satiety, while quinoa provides protein and fiber to keep you feeling full.

Vegetable Stir-Fry with Tofu:

Stir-fry a mix of colorful vegetables such as bell peppers, broccoli, snap peas, carrots, and mushrooms in a wok or skillet with a small amount of sesame oil and soy sauce. Add cubed tofu for plant-based protein and texture. Serve the vegetable stir-fry over cooked brown rice or cauliflower rice for a filling and nutritious dinner that's low in calories and high in fiber. Customize the stir-fry with your favorite vegetables and seasonings for endless flavor variations.

Turkey and Quinoa Stuffed Bell Peppers:

Prepare a filling mixture of cooked quinoa, lean ground turkey, diced tomatoes, black beans, corn, onions, garlic, and spices such as cumin, chili powder, and paprika. Stuff the mixture into halved bell peppers and bake in the oven until the peppers are tender and the filling is heated through. Top with shredded cheese and fresh cilantro for extra flavor. These stuffed bell peppers are packed with protein, fiber, and nutrients, making them a satisfying and wholesome dinner option for weight loss.

Zucchini Noodles with Turkey Meatballs:

Spiralize zucchini into noodles and sauté in a skillet with olive oil and minced garlic until tender. Meanwhile,

prepare lean turkey meatballs seasoned with Italian herbs and spices. Serve the zucchini noodles with turkey meatballs and marinara sauce for a lighter and lower-carb alternative to traditional pasta. This dinner is high in protein and fiber, yet low in calories, making it perfect for satisfying cravings while supporting weight loss efforts.
Vegetarian Chili with Sweet Potato:

Make a hearty vegetarian chili using a mix of beans such as black beans, kidney beans, and chickpeas, along with diced tomatoes, onions, bell peppers, corn, and spices such as chili powder, cumin, and smoked paprika. Add cubed sweet potatoes for sweetness and texture. Simmer the chili on the stove until thick and flavorful. Serve with a dollop of Greek yogurt or avocado slices for added creaminess. This vegetarian chili is packed with fiber and protein, making it a filling and satisfying dinner option for weight loss.
Baked Chicken Parmesan with Spaghetti Squash:

Bread chicken breasts in whole-wheat breadcrumbs seasoned with Italian herbs and spices. Bake in the oven until crispy and golden brown. Meanwhile, roast spaghetti squash until tender and scrape out the flesh into strands. Serve the baked chicken Parmesan over spaghetti squash noodles with marinara sauce and a sprinkle of Parmesan cheese. This lighter version of a classic Italian dish is lower in calories and carbs, yet still satisfying and flavorful.
Lentil and Vegetable Soup:

Make a hearty lentil and vegetable soup using green or brown lentils, diced tomatoes, carrots, celery, onions, garlic, and spices such as thyme, bay leaves, and parsley. Simmer the soup on the stove until the lentils are tender and the flavors have melded together. Serve with a slice of whole-grain bread or a side salad for a complete and satisfying meal. This soup is high in fiber and protein, making it a filling and nutritious option for weight loss.

These satisfying dinner ideas are not only delicious and nutritious but also support your weight loss goals by providing balanced meals that keep you feeling full and satisfied. By incorporating lean proteins, fiber-rich vegetables, and whole grains into your dinners, you can enjoy satisfying meals while working towards your weight loss goals.

Guilt-Free Snacks and Desserts:

When it comes to satisfying cravings for snacks and desserts while maintaining a healthy lifestyle, it's all about balance and moderation. Enjoying guilt-free treats that are lower in calories, sugar, and unhealthy fats can help you satisfy your sweet tooth and curb cravings without derailing your progress. Here are some delicious and nutritious guilt-free snacks and desserts to enjoy:

Guilt-Free Snacks:

Greek Yogurt with Fresh Fruit:

Enjoy a serving of Greek yogurt topped with fresh berries, sliced bananas, or diced mango for a creamy and satisfying snack that's rich in protein, calcium, and vitamins. Greek yogurt provides probiotics that support gut health, while the fruit adds natural sweetness and fiber.
Vegetable Sticks with Hummus:

Dip crunchy vegetable sticks such as carrots, cucumbers, bell peppers, and celery into creamy hummus for a satisfying and nutritious snack that's packed with fiber, vitamins, and minerals. Hummus provides protein and healthy fats, while the vegetables add crunch and hydration.

Air-Popped Popcorn:

Enjoy a bowl of air-popped popcorn seasoned with a sprinkle of nutritional yeast, smoked paprika, or garlic powder for a satisfying and low-calorie snack that's high in fiber and whole grains. Popcorn is a whole-food snack that provides volume without excess calories, making it a guilt-free option for satisfying cravings.
Mixed Nuts and Dried Fruit:

Create your own trail mix by combining a mix of raw or lightly salted nuts such as almonds, walnuts, and cashews with dried fruit such as raisins, apricots, and cranberries. Portion out individual servings for a convenient and satisfying snack that provides a balance of protein, healthy fats, and carbohydrates.
Rice Cake with Nut Butter:

Spread almond butter, peanut butter, or sunflower seed butter onto a rice cake for a crunchy and satisfying snack that's rich in protein, healthy fats, and fiber. Top with sliced bananas, apple slices, or berries for added sweetness and flavor.
Guilt-Free Desserts:

Frozen Yogurt Bark:

Spread Greek yogurt onto a baking sheet lined with parchment paper and top with fresh fruit, nuts, seeds, and a drizzle of honey or maple syrup. Freeze until firm,

then break into pieces for a refreshing and nutritious dessert that's low in calories and high in protein.
Chocolate Avocado Pudding:

Blend ripe avocados with unsweetened cocoa powder, a splash of almond milk, vanilla extract, and a natural sweetener such as dates or honey until smooth and creamy. Chill in the refrigerator until firm, then serve topped with shaved dark chocolate or fresh berries for a decadent and healthy dessert option.
Baked Apple Slices with Cinnamon:

Slice apples thinly and arrange on a baking sheet. Sprinkle with cinnamon and bake in the oven until tender and caramelized. Serve warm with a dollop of Greek yogurt or a sprinkle of granola for a comforting and guilt-free dessert that's naturally sweet and satisfying.
Chia Seed Pudding:

Mix chia seeds with your choice of milk (such as almond milk, coconut milk, or dairy milk) and a natural sweetener such as maple syrup or agave nectar. Let the mixture sit in the refrigerator until thickened, then serve topped with fresh fruit, nuts, seeds, or shredded coconut for a nutritious and filling dessert option.
Frozen Banana Bites:

Slice ripe bananas into rounds and dip them in melted dark chocolate. Place on a baking sheet lined with parchment paper and freeze until firm. Enjoy these bite-sized treats straight from the freezer for a sweet and satisfying dessert that's rich in potassium and antioxidants.

By incorporating these guilt-free snacks and desserts into your daily routine, you can satisfy cravings and indulge in treats without compromising your health and wellness goals. Remember to practice portion control and mindful eating to fully enjoy these delicious and nutritious treats while maintaining balance in your diet.

8. Conclusion

In conclusion, achieving and maintaining a healthy weight is not just about counting calories or following restrictive diets. It's about making sustainable lifestyle changes that promote overall well-being and support long-term success. By focusing on nutritious, balanced meals, regular physical activity, and mindful eating habits, you can reach your weight loss goals while still enjoying delicious and satisfying food.

Throughout this guide, we've explored various aspects of weight loss, from understanding the science behind it to overcoming common challenges and developing healthy habits. We've provided practical tips, delicious recipes, and meal planning strategies to help you navigate your weight loss journey with confidence and ease.

Remember that progress takes time and patience, and it's important to celebrate every small victory along the way. Whether it's choosing a nutritious snack over a sugary treat or sticking to your workout routine despite a busy schedule, every positive choice brings you closer to your goals.

Above all, be kind to yourself and listen to your body's cues. Honor your hunger and fullness, practice self-care, and seek support from friends, family, or a healthcare professional when needed. By prioritizing your health and well-being, you can create a sustainable lifestyle that allows you to thrive physically, mentally, and emotionally.

Here's to your continued success on your weight loss journey. May you find joy, fulfillment, and balance in every step you take towards a healthier, happier you.

Celebrating Your Progress:

As you embark on your weight loss journey, it's important to acknowledge and celebrate the progress you make along the way. Celebrating your achievements, no matter how small, can provide motivation, boost confidence, and reinforce positive behaviors. Here are some meaningful ways to celebrate your progress:

Set Milestones: Break your weight loss journey into smaller, manageable goals or milestones. Whether it's losing a certain number of pounds, fitting into a smaller clothing size, or achieving a fitness milestone, celebrate each achievement as a stepping stone towards your ultimate goal.

Reward Yourself: Treat yourself to non-food rewards when you reach a milestone or achieve a goal. Choose rewards that align with your interests and values, such as buying a new workout outfit, booking a massage, or indulging in a spa day. These rewards serve as reminders of your hard work and dedication.

Reflect on Your Successes: Take time to reflect on your progress and accomplishments. Keep a journal or log of your achievements, milestones, and positive experiences throughout your weight loss journey.

Reviewing your successes can boost confidence and motivation during challenging times.

Share Your Successes: Share your progress and successes with supportive friends, family members, or online communities. Celebrating your achievements with others not only reinforces your commitment to your goals but also allows you to receive encouragement and support from those who care about your well-being.

Document Your Journey: Document your weight loss journey through photos, journal entries, or blog posts. Take progress photos regularly to visually track your transformation over time. Looking back on how far you've come can be incredibly rewarding and motivating.

Celebrate Non-Scale Victories: Celebrate achievements that go beyond the number on the scale. Recognize improvements in energy levels, mood, fitness, strength, and overall well-being. These non-scale victories are just as important as weight loss and deserve to be celebrated.

Plan a Celebration Meal or Activity: Plan a special meal or activity to celebrate reaching a significant milestone in your weight loss journey. Choose a healthy yet indulgent meal at your favorite restaurant or plan a fun outdoor adventure such as hiking, biking, or kayaking with friends or family.

Practice Gratitude: Take a moment to express gratitude for your body and the progress you've made. Focus on the positive changes you've experienced and the habits you've cultivated along the way. Practicing gratitude can shift your perspective and enhance feelings of satisfaction and contentment.

By celebrating your progress and achievements, you acknowledge the hard work and dedication you've invested in your health and well-being. Embrace each milestone as a testament to your strength, resilience, and commitment to living your best life. Remember that every step forward, no matter how small, brings you closer to your goals and a happier, healthier you.

Maintaining Your Weight Loss Journey:

Congratulations on reaching your weight loss goals! Now that you've achieved success, it's time to focus on maintaining your progress and embracing a healthy lifestyle for the long term. Maintaining weight loss can be just as challenging as losing weight, but with the right strategies and mindset, you can sustain your achievements and continue to thrive. Here are some tips for maintaining your weight loss journey:

Establish Sustainable Habits: Focus on incorporating sustainable habits into your daily routine that support your health and well-being. This includes eating a balanced diet rich in fruits, vegetables, lean proteins, and whole grains, staying hydrated, getting regular physical activity, prioritizing sleep, managing stress, and practicing mindful eating.

Monitor Your Progress: Continue to monitor your weight and measurements regularly to track your progress and catch any changes early on. This can help you stay accountable and make adjustments to your lifestyle as needed to maintain your weight loss.

Stay Active: Physical activity is essential for weight maintenance and overall health. Aim for at least 150 minutes of moderate-intensity aerobic exercise or 75 minutes of vigorous-intensity aerobic exercise each week, along with muscle-strengthening activities on two or more days per week. Find activities you enjoy and make them a regular part of your routine.

Practice Portion Control: Be mindful of portion sizes and practice portion control to prevent overeating. Use smaller plates and bowls, measure out serving sizes, and pay attention to hunger and fullness cues. Focus on eating slowly and savoring each bite to fully enjoy your meals.

Keep Healthy Foods Accessible: Stock your kitchen with healthy, nutrient-dense foods that support your weight maintenance goals. Keep fresh fruits and vegetables, lean proteins, whole grains, and healthy snacks readily available for quick and convenient meals and snacks.

Plan Ahead: Plan your meals and snacks in advance to avoid impulsive or unhealthy choices. Create a weekly meal plan, make a grocery list, and prep ingredients ahead of time to streamline mealtime and reduce the temptation to rely on convenience foods or takeout.

Stay Hydrated: Drink plenty of water throughout the day to stay hydrated and support your body's functions. Choose water as your primary beverage and limit sugary drinks, alcohol, and high-calorie beverages. Staying hydrated can help prevent overeating and support overall health.

Practice Self-Care: Prioritize self-care activities that promote relaxation, stress management, and emotional well-being. Take time for activities you enjoy, such as reading, gardening, practicing yoga, or spending time with loved ones. Managing stress and prioritizing self-care can help prevent emotional eating and support weight maintenance.

Stay Flexible: Be flexible and adaptable with your approach to weight maintenance. Life is unpredictable, and there will be times when your routine is disrupted or you face challenges. Instead of striving for perfection, focus on progress and making healthy choices most of the time.

Seek Support: Surround yourself with a supportive network of friends, family, or a community who understand your goals and can provide encouragement, accountability, and motivation. Share your successes and challenges with others, and celebrate your achievements together.

Remember that maintaining weight loss is a lifelong journey that requires commitment, consistency, and self-awareness. By incorporating these strategies into your daily life and staying focused on your health and well-being, you can continue to thrive and enjoy the benefits of your hard work for years to come. Here's to a happy, healthy, and fulfilling future ahead!

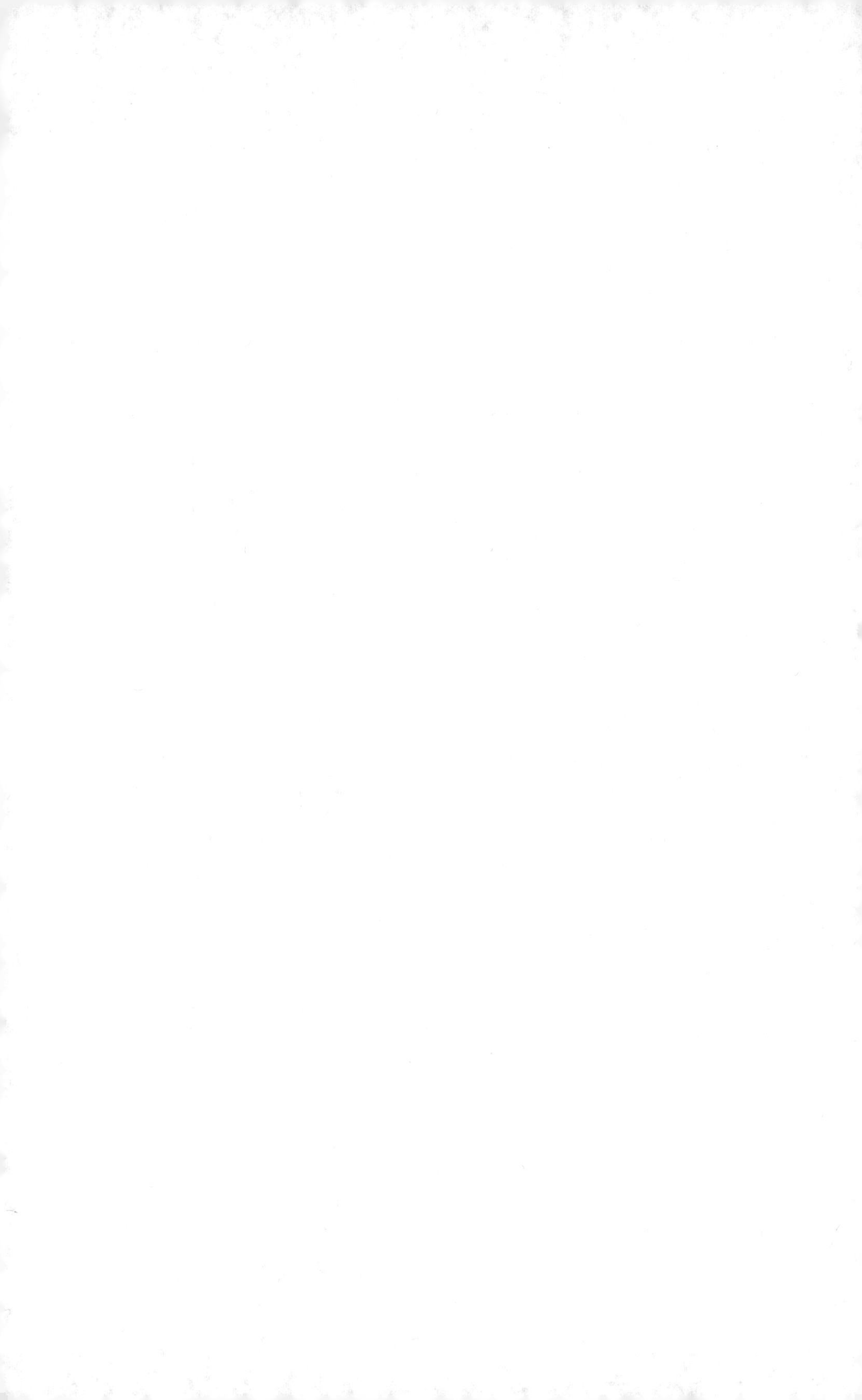